CW00497372

No Rhyme or Reason

Paul Martin

Edward Gaskell *publishers*
DEVON

First published 2008
Edward Gaskell *publishers*
The Old *Gazette* Building
6 Grenville Street
Bideford
Devon
EX39 2EA

isbn(10) 1-906769-03-6
    (13) 978-1-906769-03-1

© Paul Martin
© Illustrations Bill Wright

No Rhyme or Reason
Paul Martin

All rights reserved. No part of this publication may be reproduced, stored in a
retrieval system, or transmitted in any form by any means electronic, mechani-
cal, photocopying, scanning, recording or otherwise, without the prior written
permission of the publishers.

Typeset, printed and bound by
Lazarus Press
Caddsdown Business Park
Bideford
Devon
EX39 3DX
www.lazaruspress.com

Contents

Edward Gaskell *publishers*
DEVON

To My Children

Lucas Max and Hattie May

Foreword

This is a fascinating and important book: not only as a collection of poetry to be enjoyed and admired, but also as a telling, sometimes shocking, reminder of the fact that Parkinson's disease can strike at almost any age. The clichéd image of the elderly, trembling man as being typical of this complex, distressing disease is firmly dispatched in this candid expression of just what it can be like to be a young person living with Parkinson's.

I've been involved with the PDS for many years now, and I am always struck by how especially tough it can be for those who are diagnosed at a young age. Anything that can help to spread awareness of the problems, thoughts and experiences of this younger age group with PD is to be welcomed, and Paul's terrific poems do just that, in a wonderfully creative and emotive way.

I'm sure his thoughts will resonate with many others and, at the same time, raise some much needed funds for the PDS, helping us to support more people living with the condition and to move ever closer to our ultimate goal of finding a cure.

Jane Asher

President Parkinson's Disease Society

Introduction

24th April 2004, this date will be etched on my mind forever. I was just 33 years old at the time and life was good. I had just started a new job, I was living with my partner Melissa, I had been blessed with a beautiful little boy and I was relishing my role as a relatively new if not slightly naïve Father. My son Lucas Max was 18 months old and at the time I can say without doubt I had never been happier. That's when my perfect world collapsed around me. I had been admitted to hospital two days earlier because I had taken a funny turn at work and it raised enough concern in my mind that on my way home I stopped at A&E. I had been having slight problems prior to this with the dexterity in the fingers on my left hand and slowness of movement in my left arm, but had not been too concerned; I just thought that I had slept on it funny or maybe even trapped a nerve. Nothing could have prepared me for the diagnosis that was to be delivered on that fateful day:

'Mr Martin you have early onset Parkinsons Disease'.

That is where my personal journey with PD started. Initially I shut it out and for the first six months I refused to let the diagnosis sink in and just tried to get on with my life. Upon reflection this head-in-the-sand approach was to be the catalyst of a serious bout of depression.

I was referred for counselling and that's when I was told that writing down how I feel both emotionally and physically would help me start to face my condition and would also help the people close to me understand what was going on in my head.

I never realised at the time that when I started to write down my thoughts they would come out in the form of poems, but for some reason they did. The poems are simple and nothing more than just rhyming couplets, I'm hardly a poet so excuse the simplicity, but they do convey my fears and emotions. They also show that although you try to stay strong and positive, one day you feel you can beat it and the next all the fear and emotions can consume you and you can very quickly start to spiral towards a bout of depression. I am sure that the content of the poems and living your life with this condition will be recognised by, and have been experienced by other sufferers, their carers and family and friends.

It's a lonely disease to live with and if reading this helps one person with this condition realise they are not alone or helps a family member or friend understand what may be going on inside their loved-one's head, then that can only be a good thing.

Welcome to my world.

Paul Martin

Acknowledgements

My thanks to Richard Hames of MDH Insurance, Bedford, for his generosity in sponsoring the printing and publishing costs of this book.

My thanks also to Bill Wright of Appledore, North Devon. A very talented artist and book illustrator who generously gave freely of his time and talent.

My family and friends without whom I would not have come through this diagnosis. Their love and support has humbled me.

Finally Debbie Blake my Parkinson's Disease Specialist Nurse. From day one she has never let me feel sorry for myself for too long. Her *get on with it* and *stop moaning* approach to my condition and her bedside manner never fail to make me smile. Debbie and the team are an invaluable resource to have to hand and they have never complained once about my million or so phone calls.

Thank you for helping me stay positive.

Yesterday

See you Monday!

This is where my story begins. When diagnosed with a devastating illness such as PD, MS, or cancer it is important to receive support and information and to have somewhere to turn to. I hope no one else when diagnosed went through the emotions and fear that I did when I was delivered my bombshell.

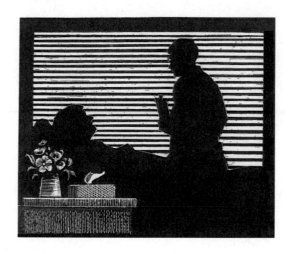

See you Monday!

Wednesday, Thursday, Friday
That is how long it took
For my life to be turned upside down
A horror story in a book

I lay there on my bed
My son was next to me
Surely I misheard him?
Mr Martin you have PD!

Surely the neuro's got it wrong
That's an illness of the old
His manner was matter of fact
His delivery somewhat cold

Will I see my son grow up?
Will I play in goal again?
Will I start to waste away?
Or will I live my life in pain?

I remember asking the questions
As I lay there in that bed
He answered, I saw his lips move
But I never heard what he said

My brain was working overtime
My body had gone numb
Little did I know then
There was more of that to come

As I said, this was on a Friday
The clock said it's nearly four
Within an hour of diagnosis
I opened my front door.

Looking back I can't get to grips
Just being sent home like this
Come back and see me Monday
Excuse me! You taking the piss?

What he had just told me
Had changed my life for good
Surely it's not 'see you Monday'
I must have misunderstood?

I spent the next few days
Scared and in suspense
Sent home with no information
Surely use your common sense

I hope that's not the norm
When diagnosing someone with PD
There must be support at that time
For that someone just like me.

No Rhyme or Reason

I am alone

This poem stems from some of my early thoughts. I was scared, uninformed and I did not think I had the strength or the courage to get through. I found strength through my family and friends and any suicidal thoughts I had at the beginning have well and truly gone.

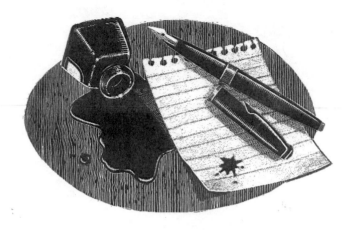

I am alone

I am alone with this paper
I clasp the pen in my hand.
I'm about to write my good-bye
About to make my last stand.

Please accept this as an apology
For turning to this knife
I cannot face what is my future
So tonight I'm taking my life

The emotions consume and overcome me
Feels like I'm swimming against the tide
I try to swim, but I get nowhere
I just can't reach the other side

You told me I could make it
Oh how I wish that you were right.
It's a struggle to get through the day
And it only gets worse at night

Sometimes I feel so defeated,
Can't find strength to get out of bed
For when I'm awake, they become real
The painful thoughts inside my head

It's just too big a battle
This dragon's too big to be slayed
I never really stood a chance
So I've had my headstone made

On my headstone it just says
'Here lies Paul he is no more
Parkinsons stole his life away
September 1970 - April 2004'

So, this is my cowardly note
It tells of my suicide
I wish I could fight through it all
But I can't, my soul has died

Despite what I have written
I am scared as hell to die
For the after-life's unknown
But I've lost the will to try

My way out lays beside me
Can I let this illness win?
Knowing that if I choose to die
I'll never know what could have been.

No Rhyme or Reason

Another baby on the way

We were on holiday at the time. We had not been planning to extend the family in the immediate future, so this news came as a shock. We had discussed whether we would have another baby after I was diagnosed, and although we knew we wanted a sibling for Lucas there was always an element of worry about having more children.

Another baby on the way

It was at the end of a beautiful day
We were all having a lark
Rubber rings and water slides
Having fun at the water park

It was then I first found out
There was something you had to say
That was the first time you told me
Another baby was on the way

You hadn't told me sooner
'Cos you knew I'd be a pain
You knew I'd start to worry
And I'd drive you all insane

At first I was so jubilant
With a smile from ear to ear
But once the news had sunk in
The excitement turned to fear

How would I manage this time?
Now I'm diagnosed with PD
Life was a lot simpler
When we had our first baby

Will I be able to change a nappy?
Can I get them ready for bed?
Will I be any kind of father?
Were some of the thoughts inside my head

The next seven months went so fast
And I could never be prepared
The thought of someone else to love
I've never been so scared

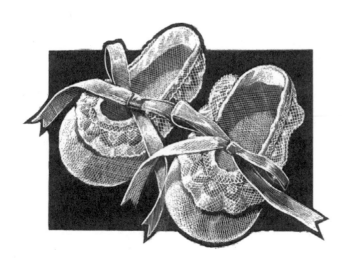

I'll always remember the day she arrived
The 3rd of January 2006
The fear had suddenly disappeared
I look so happy in the pics

I was blessed with a daughter
On that winter's day
The day I was sent my princess
The very beautiful Hattie May

But the smiles didn't last
And it wasn't very long
Before people started to realise
That something was very wrong

I started to resent her being here
She was getting in the way
I just wanted my time with Lucas
'Post-natal depression', I heard someone say

I lost my mind and left
Just left it all behind
Sitting for months in my flat
Going out of my mind

One night I was dreaming
And the Devil came to me
And offered me a deal
He'd swop my children for my PD

When I woke up that morning
And lay there in my bed
I reflected on my dream that night
And what the Devil said

I realised that morning
I wasn't the important one
The only ones that were important
Were my daughter and my son

I went back to sleep to meet the Devil
I had something I had to tell
Swop my children for PD?
Lucifer you can go to hell

I'll love you every single day
And make you proud of me
And if ever given the choice again
Then I would always choose PD

I'm so glad to have you Hattie
And I want to shout out loud
That you're funny, cute and beautiful
And you make Daddy so very proud.

Your hero once again

One of my worries when I was first diagnosed was would my children ever feel embarrased by me. Would my son want me at the sideline cheering him on or would either of them be embarrased to invite their friends round for tea? I always wanted my son to see me as his hero and be proud to call me Dad.

Your hero once again

You two are the reason
I've found to stay alive
The strength to try harder
To come out the other side

I think a lot to myself
During the sleepless nights
I try to come to terms with
'Why me? Why take my life?'

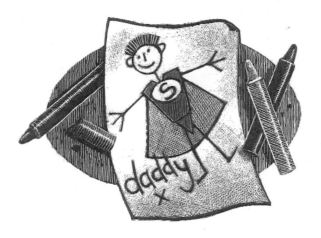

I'm not reaching out to you
Looking for your sympathy
I just hope when you are older
You can still be proud of me

I would be lost without you
You two are my guiding light
Showing me there is a future
And you make that future bright

I know there will be a cure one day
They have assured me of this
But please God in my lifetime
That is my only wish

But even when they manage
To put this wrong right
Because of you it will only be
The third best day of my life

And as they eagerly search
For that illusive pot of gold
There is just one thing I cling to
One dream I lovingly hold

I dream of a PD-free future
I pray that that these clever men
Can cure me of this illness
And I can be your hero once again

You are the very reason
I just don't let go
The reason to keep on smiling
When the pain begins to show

You both are my salvation
You protect me with your love
You help me get through the bad days
When I've really had enough

So I'm sorry for the days
When I ever let you down
I'm sorry 'cos I can't always
Joke around and play the clown

I hope one day you'll understand
Why this clown was sad from day to day
I couldn't always paint a face on
And pretend that everything's ok

I promised myself years ago
I'd try and be the perfect Dad
It's frustration, not you my babies
That makes me shout when I am mad

I think I'm the luckiest man alive
'But that's madness', I hear them say
But then they're not the Daddy
Of Lucas Max and Hattie May

You are my rays of sunshine
My little droplets of rain
I hope one day you'll see me
As your hero once again.

Changeable place

In May 2006 I embarked on a journey that would ultimately change my life. I took up the challenge to trek across the Namib Desert to help raise funds for the PDS. I was joined by my brother Nick and my friend Nick (Aka the lesser spotted ginger Albino) I can't explain how amazing this experience turned out to be. To coin a phrase: 'you had to be there'. Nick (my brother) captures it well in this poem he wrote about our adventure.

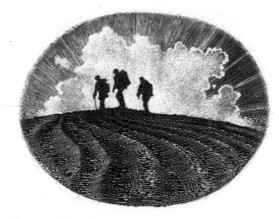

Changeable place

We spent a week in a foreign land
Where most of us were expecting sand
It soon became clear that this was not case
As we started our trek in this changeable place
The sights and the sounds were there to behold
And memories were made that will never go cold
I thought that someone was calling my bluff
But we never quite knew when enough was enough
From mountains and rivers to spine tingling shivers
United we stood as our hearts we delivered
We shared emotions in and outside our tents
The time that we spent felt like dreams I'd been lent
But now that we're back on familiar ground
I know in myself that my spirit I found
This trip that we shared will forever live on
The desert preserving how brightly we shone
So let's keep our minds and our heads in the sky
And remember the tears that fell down from our eyes
As we recount the people and places we met
On our PDS journey that we'll never forget

Frustration

It was not just my life that was turned upside down by the early onset of PD. My partner has to deal with this too and during the times when I am low or I'm struggling with it all a lot of stress and pressure is put on her. Relationships are hard work anyway, add to that the stress, worry and uncertainty that this illness brings and it becomes even harder. This poem reflects on a period in our relationship when not only was I dealing with the daily symptoms, I was going through a change in medication and at the same time I had got shingles. I was not in good shape and our relationship was facing its hardest test to date. One thing that I have learned from this is, that diagnosed with this condition, it was not just me that became a PD sufferer.

Frustration

I'm still so glad I met you
'Cos on that drunken night
I chose the mother of my children
And I got my choice just right

They are lucky to be blessed
With a mummy just like you
And I thank you from my heart
For everything you do

I thank you for the time you spend
Nurturing them everyday
The way you're always there for them
In every single way

But I find it a little frustrating
You're so perfect in this way
But you can make me so unhappy
With the hurtful things you say

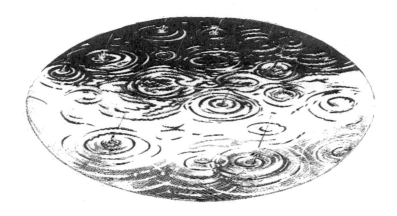

I know I'm far from perfect
And life is never always bliss
But I am human and have feelings
So do I really deserve this?

I know you never signed up
For what the future has in store
It breaks my heart you think I let you down
I just wish I could offer you more

But I never signed up either
And I feel some anger too
And I try my very hardest
Not to take it out on you

I try so hard to please you
But it never is enough
You seem so bitter towards me
Do you have to be so tough?

Despite all this I love you
And I'm glad that night I went to town
But this illness is not my fault
And I'm sad you feel I've let you down

The road ahead is a rocky one
The future's not very clear
You said everyone would be better off
If I wasn't here

I died a little inside on the
Day you said that you see
You made my life seem worthless
That you thought so little of me

I have to try so hard
To stay strong everyday
But you make it so much harder
With the hurtful things you say

I'm scared of what's in store
Of what I will become
Will I be a dissapointment
To my daughter and my son?

I can't do this without you
I need you along for the ride
But I don't need you on my back
I need you by my side.

Ginger Nick

When you have a life that is filled with constantly mixed emotions you need an outlet and a means of expressing those feelings. Poems are one way, but to have a friend who is always there is just as important. Lots of friends would let you talk, but are they listening? I know that when I'm talking Nick is listening. I do not imagine Nick really understands how important he has been since my diagnosis, but why would he? He is just being himself, a genuine guy and a true friend.

Thank you.

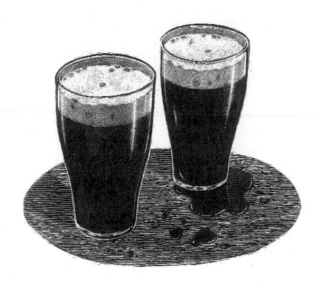

Ginger Nick

I'd like to introduce you
To this fella that I know
Referred to, by me sometimes
As the Ginger Albino

There are very few people in life
You can really call a friend
Someone who's always there for you
Time and time again

Nick is one of those people
I can count on every day
Always there to listen to me
When there is something I want to say

Nothing's ever too much trouble
He's always been there for me
Helped me on my bad days
And he has done it so willingly

He is filled with many qualities
He is caring, honest and true
And I would be more than happy
If my son grew up to be like you

We have shared good times together
We have shared some bad times too
And I thank him for being there
'Cos he helped me to pull through

We talk a lot and cry at times
About the loss of his dear mum
I'm proud to have you as a friend
As was she to have you as a son

So if you ever need me mate
There's nothing I wouldn't do
I will always be your wing man
And gladly take a bullet for you.

Today

I walk alone and I'm already dead

Today my emotions are more on the happy-go-lucky side, but that doesn't mean that it's roses all the way. Sometimes you have a bad day and the smiles are gone and the whirlwind of emotions consume you again.

The following two poems were written on the same day. It shows that emotions and moods can swing drastically from positive to negative. This does not necessarily happen over a period of time.

One minute life's great and in the next moment one negative thought occurs or something happens that makes you think too much, and 'bang' you're down again.

I walk alone

I walk alone this lonely road
As my life passes me by
I continue to walk, the path of my dreams
As the sun glistens in the sky

My memories are logged in my brain
Happiness and sadness they hold
But my body is getting tired
I'm growing up and I'm getting old

I'm no longer a little boy
Now I'm older and wiser than most
Many heartaches have ruined the past
And PD is the latest ghost

My life is now a lonely road
And I'm walking it all day long
But I'll forget the sorrow from yesterday
And I'll keep on going strong

I'll walk with a smile on my face
I'll walk with a gigantic stride
Nothing will keep me from reaching my goal
While I still carry these dreams inside.

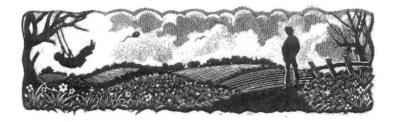

I'm already dead

The thoughts that I have
As I lay in this bed
What's the point in trying
When you're already dead?

I'm lonely and hurt,
And broken I remain
Residing in this hell,
Living with this pain

I'm doomed by this illness
As I slowly fade away
The nightmare that I live with
Each and every day

The meaning of it all
To which my mind attends
But no one has an answer
That I fully comprehend

I go out of my mind
I want a cure for us all,
They keep reaching for it
But it's a never-ending fall

'Stay strong and keep going
There'll be a cure', you all say
But no-one seems to realize
The pain I suffer every day

There's no such thing as help
Outside of your mind
It's you against yourself
With your demons intertwined

It's a battle, hard fought
But never to be won
Either way you end up losing
When it's all said and done

'Too late' came and passed
And, of me, nothing more
I wrote my own ending
And I shut my own door

'Live your life to its fullest,'
That's what they all said
But what's the point in trying
When you're already dead?

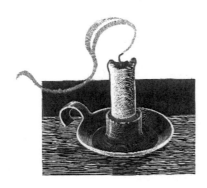

I'm just like Elvis

Not a prize winner this one but it made me see that before I was diagnosed I actually never realised how happy I was and that I had everything that really made me happy.

Shame that it took this illness to make me realise that.

I'm just like Elvis

My life is just like Elvis'
I know that's hard to comprehend
We both had everything we wanted
Then it was all brought to an end

When growing up he was my idol
And it's crazy to be compared
But our lives were similar I think
And a lot of things we shared

The comparison is very obscure
We liked junk food and girls alike
He was a Rock and Roll legend
And I was just the village bike

He had all that he could dream of
All the money and the fame
I also felt I'd won the pools
And to me that's just the same

Because I had been blessed
With two little bundles of joy
One was a beautiful little girl
The other a gorgeous little boy

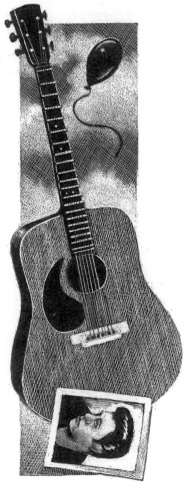

It's hard to accept your life
When you feel you've won the cup
And then just like Elvis's life
An illness f***s it up

I hope that's where the comparison stops
And the similarity comes to an end
'Cos I wouldn't want to be found dead
On the bog by a family friend.

Good Morning

It is hard to imagine how it feels as you slowly watch and see the changes that you go through as the condition progresses. Such straight forward exercises and daily rituals that we take for granted become tasks in themselves. This is the start to my typical morning.

Good Morning

I awake in the morning
The working day ahead
I've had very little sleep
But I must get out of bed

I am like an old man
As I shuffle across the floor
Muscles already beginning to ache
Before I reach the bedroom door

I walk to the bathroom on tip toe
There is a cramp in my calf
To get my body moving
It's another bloody bath

Such an effort to get dry
But this is nothing new
Frustrating, something so simple
Has become so difficult to do

By the time I put my clothes on
And before I've even fed
My body is so tired
And wants to get back in the bed

Time to go down stairs
Already full of frustration
Here comes the first dose
Of my daily medication

Lucas and Hattie are having breakfast
They bring a smile to my face
They really keep me going
And are my saving grace

It's so hard to stay smiling
'Cos every morning is the same
I feel like I've done a day's work
'It's a funny old game'

By eight my head is spinning
My emotions are going berserk
I feel like it's time for bed
But it's only time for work.

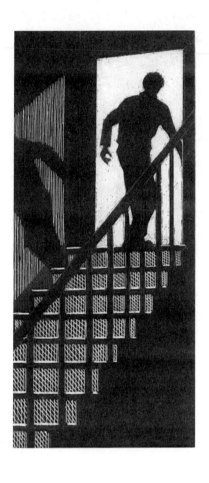

The field of dreams

As previously mentioned I spend a lot of time in the bath, sometimes the muscle rigidity and slowness of movement are quite uncomfortable. This is relieved immensely by immersing myself in a steaming hot bath. This not only relaxes the body but also the mind. When I take my morning soak it's quite early and as I lie there, with my eyes closed, dawn arrives and the birds break into song. It's peaceful and very relaxing. . . I'd recommend all to start your stressful days like this. We all have a field of dreams somewhere.

Anyway, this poem stems from these early morning soaks.

The field of dreams

I found myself lying there
In a field of my own dreams
Enjoying the sun that shone
And the joys that life brings

I lay with my eyes closed
Dreaming without a care
I felt like I could touch the clouds
As if I were really there

I could reach out and touch them
As if they were real
And could smell the flowers
Even touch how they feel

I could hear the birds waking
What sounds they would bring
From one bird to another
In harmony they would sing

Suddenly there was a silence
From this path I'd strayed
Then the sound of running water
Of the stream not far away

As I turned to look behind me
I began then to realize
My field of dreams had faded away
I must have opened my eyes

If I hear a running stream
Or birds begin to sing
I close my eyes and I am there
I'm in the field of dreams.

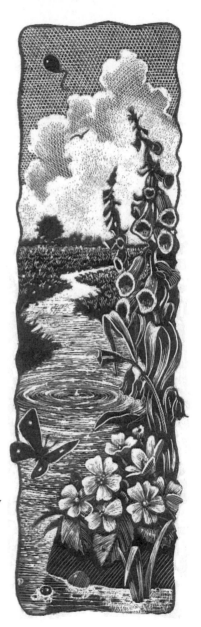

Rollercoaster

Definition:

1. A steep, sharply curving, elevated railway with small open passenger cars that is operated at high speed as a ride, especially in an amusement park.

2. An action, event, or experience marked by abrupt, extreme changes in circumstance, quality, or behaviour.

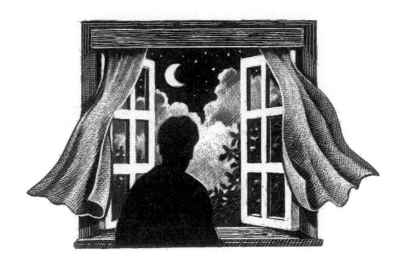

Rollercoaster

Another night with no sleep
Tossing from side to side
Desperately trying to nod off
My mind's in overdrive

I lay there for hours on end
Trying to shut down my brain
But once it gets going, it's off
It's like a runaway train

I think a lot about my children
And one thing fills me with dread
What happens when I can't work
How will I keep a roof over their head?

This is the time I have to be careful
When my mind starts getting stressed
It's when I feel most vulnerable
And a sign that I'm getting depressed

I have to try to stay positive
But it's hard, believe me I've tried
So the only thing to do is hold tight
'Cos it's a rollercoaster ride

I could let my emotions run away
And just live life in despair
And just stay on this rollercoaster
Which is neither fun nor fair

But if I let my emotions run away
And if I let them take control
Then I've let this disease win
And to the Devil I've sold my soul

So when I visit the theme park
And I'm on that rollercoaster ride
I'll smile and laugh and have fun
With my children by my side.

No Rhyme or Reason

I choose life

I'm at the point now where this is it! I've got it, there's absolutely nothing I can do about it. If I let it control me today it's won. As I see it, it's got my future, it never had my past and if I don't let it win today then I'm in the lead. Me 2 - Parkinsons 1

I choose life

Sometimes I wish I could look at the world
Through rose-coloured specs
So I see the good things in life
And not just see the negatives

Pain is a part of my life
But I do choose to live
Life's about more than just surviving
It's about what you have to give

Living is so much more
Than just being alive
It's a willingness to want
A willingness to strive

Hiding away from the pain
If in self pity you immerse
You're only hiding from reality
And can only make things worse

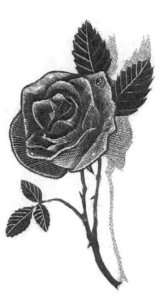

So live life to its fullest
That's what living life should be
To live life with a passion
And play the hand life dealt to me

Pain is a part of my life
But there is also happiness
Living life only for the pain
Would be a life of emptiness

I will live life to its fullest
And give it all I have to give
'Cos what's the point in being alive
If you're not prepared to live?

Happy Birthday

These times of the year are what still get me, birth-days and Christmas etc. I have always struggled to deal with the emotions, fear and uncertainty I feel around the time of these annual events. But, I will enjoy my birthday this year! Last year I had never written a poem, this year I'm having a book of poems published. What an amazing year. Next year? Bring it on.

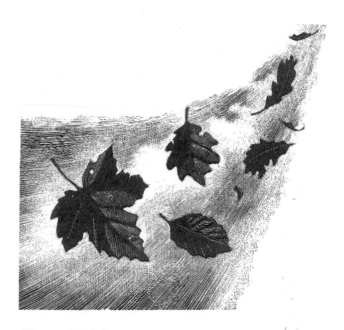

Happy Birthday

It's nearing that time again
The time to celebrate
Spiralling towards the big four 'o'
And this year I'm thirty-eight

It's supposed to be a happy time
A good time in your life
And believe me I am happy
But it's a double-edged knife

On one hand I am happy
On the other hand it's a curse
Reflecting on how I was last year, and now
And wondering if next year I'll be worse?

It's the same on all occasions
That come round each and every year
Thinking about yesterday, today, tomorrow
And that's why I'll shed a tear

So on my birthday you might see me smiling
But you'll know if I'm looking down
I'm thinking about yesterday, today, tomorrow
So please excuse the forlorn frown.

Tomorrow

Tomorrow

Enough Said.

Tomorrow

This is the only poem in here
'Cos tomorrow's a dream away
And you can't worry about tomorrow
If you're living for today

It cannot be about tomorrow
If I write it down today
I know that sounds a bit weird
But tomorrow today will be yesterday

Let's not worry about tomorrow
When there's so much to do today
There're things to do and people to see,
While the sun shines, let's make hay

So all I'll say about the future
Is I hope they find the solution
And put an end to the mystery
Is it environmental or gene mutation?

All you need to know about tomorrow
Is in the very last verse
'Cos they'll finally crack the riddle
And they'll exorcise this curse

And when they find that pot of gold
At the end of the rainbow
We can enjoy today so much more
And look forward to tomorrow.

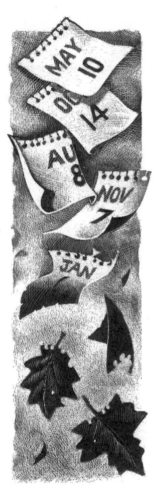

Lazarus Press
DEVON